Hello

Hello Beautiful!

I dedicate this book of weight management and beauty to you.
Because I was thinking of you when I wrote this book.

The day you were born was a special day. The Earth was a better
place and that hasn't changed. I want to thank you for who you are
because without you, someone in this world would not be loved.
You were born to bring color, kindness, comfort and strength.

This book is about helping you become the vibrant woman you
were meant to be.

You can change and I can teach you how.

Welcome to GLOW. You're entering into a journey of
transformation, a path that together over the next 12 months
will help you to find the beauty that comes from a genuine
love of your womanhood. It's a path of dreamers and if
you choose to embrace it, you will emerge your best self.
This journey of self-discovery is a game changer. It's
exciting to think of your ultimate destiny.

Now let's begin.

1 You Have To Add Before You Subtract

You thought this was a weight-loss book, huh? Maybe behavior modification? Really, it's more than that. Or should I say better?

I'm going to add to your life; you may find that you feel fuller than ever before. You don't believe me, do you? You decide.

One more thing. If you are already on a weight loss program, you can choose to stay on it. Whatever you are doing, my plan will make it far more effective.

It Always Starts with Water

You're already drinking eight glasses a day? That's amazing! I want you to do something for me. Add in one can (12 fluid ounces or 355 milligrams) of sparkling water.

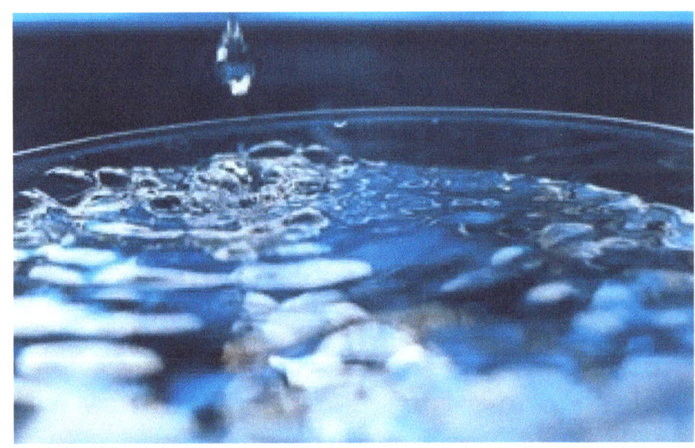

As for those of you who say, "Oops, I'm not drinking eight glasses of water," I say "Great! Don't start." Just add one can of sparkling water to your day.

Congratulation! That's Day 1.

For the next six days, drink one can of sparkling
water. That's Week One. What do you think of it?
Did you put ice in it? Lemon or lime? Did you drink
it at room temperature or however you did it, this is
the beginning of a new you!

Now, if you've gotten to this part of the book, I'll
tell you why I added one can of sparkling water to
your life. Because French girls do it. The French
like it easy. I just figured you would, too.

This is what you just did: You lost 100 calories for a
glass of soda or fruit juice and you also cut down up
to one-sixth of any meal because you filled your
stomach with air as well as water, causing you to
feel fuller with every sip.

Now you do the math. One-sixth of any meal could
be anywhere from 120 calories to 300 calories. Add
in the 100 calories you didn't drink in soda, you just
subtract 220 – 400 calories from any meal.

Multiply than by three meals in a day and you've
avoided 660 to 1,200 calories a day.

So now, you decide – and only you can – if you

want to add another can of soda water to your life.
As it stands, you'll save 1,400 calories per week,
one and one-third pounds a month from the little
itty bitty can.

What would happen if you added four cans a day
and changed nothing else? That's four and a half
pounds per month that you don't gain but lose
instead.

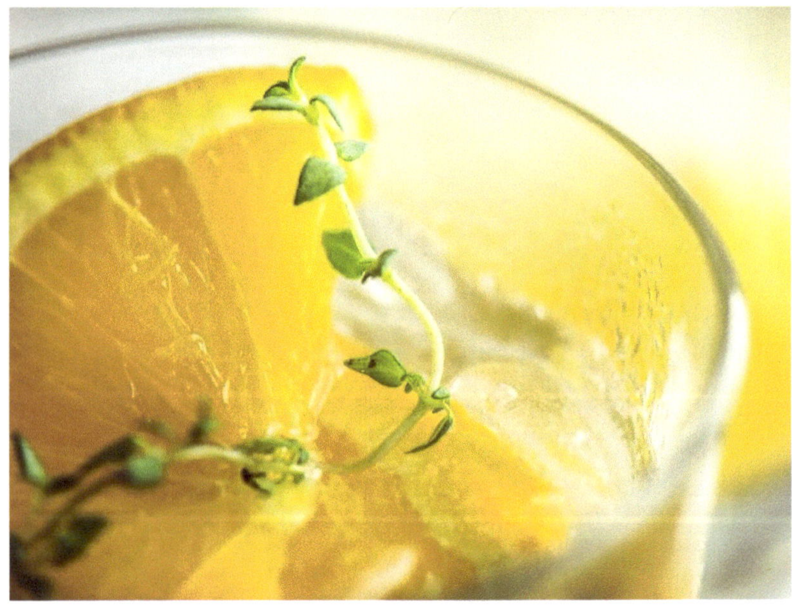

Add the History of Sparkling Water?}

Garcinia Cambrosia?

Feel free to try it! But if you're like me, I will just put some lemon in your water. They both provide the same metabolic boost. It's just that lemons are cheaper, more readily available and they taste better. This is a proven method of Greek and Italian women who have to stay bikini ready. It will work for you too if you care to add it to all your water or your salad or even your soups.

Please avoid drinking spoonfuls of lemon juice. Add it to your food or drink instead. It's a flavor boost, not a potion. It also helps you liven up dishes and need less salt to cook with.

It's a win/win, folks! You are well on your way.

Would you like to learn more? Add an apple or a banana just before you eat. Pair it with your can of soda water. Eat it with your breakfast and eat it before your lunch or dinner. If you find yourself feeling a little full, eat what you can of your meals and feel free to box up the rest if you're at a restaurant – tomorrow's lunch!

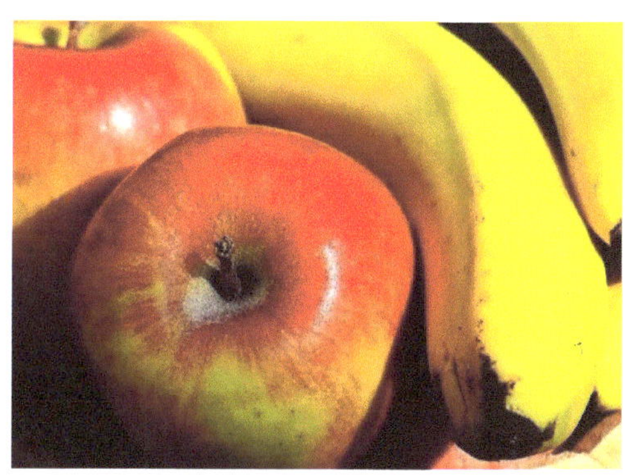

Or you can opt for less if you're at home or pack lunch.

I got you! You don't think it's gonna work? 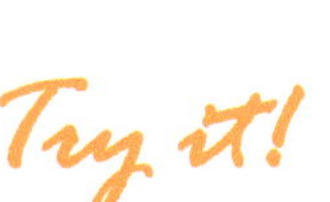

That's Month One. Are you excited? Well? What does excite you? Whatever does excite you, you need energy to enjoy it. And I do believe this month will leave you feeling more energetic and enthusiastic – about yourself and the things you love to do and the people you love to do them with.

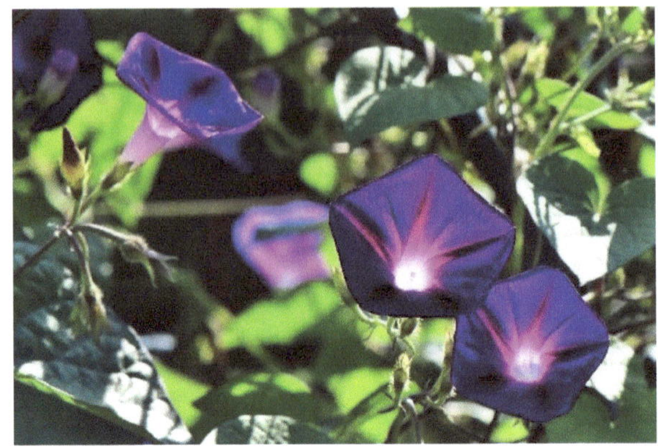

Once you find yourself five pounds lighter, add in some movement. Now, add in a walk for 30 minutes. It doesn't need to be all together. You can park further away from the grocery store. Add to that some stairs at work; turn on some music and dance, do a video, take a class. Just as long as it adds up to 30 minutes every other day.

There's no limit to the things you can do to get moving, but I recommend the Dunn's book, ***Put on Your Shoes and Take that Walk*** because it's all about getting started today! If you wanna do something more exciting tomorrow or creative, have at it.

Talk to you later!

So proud of you!

2 Why Gift Wrap It?

This is a key principle of this book. Do this and you will be well on your way to the body you desire.

So what does the term "gift wrap it" mean? It's a little-known technique used by women in India. I consider it to be one of the most valuable pieces of information I gleaned from my college education. The premise is this: When young women have a baby, their mother or aunts would wrap cloth tightly around their waist. The result would be a return to their pre-pregnancy figure.

I have found this to be one of the key features in achieving a slim waist line.

Rather than wrapping cloth, I recommend using a girdle. Check with your doctor first to find if it is right for you.

Do not use this method if you have chronic health issues such as high blood pressure, kidney failure or digestive problems. Please consult your doctor first.

Remember, as you lose weight, discard your larger clothes. Take this time to study color. Look for such books as ***Color Me Beautiful.*** Also, consider getting a subscription to a fashion magazine. The more you wear clothing that looks good on you, the better you will feel. Don't wait for that final weight goal …

Dress yourself well now!

3 Use it or Lose it

You have a beautiful body.

It was perfectly deigned and perfectly knit together in your mother's womb. It is a precious gift and you should be happy with it. But so many of us are not happy with our bodies. Why? Because we have been living unnatural lifestyles that include long periods of inactivity like sitting in a chair for hours in an office. This keeps the body in an unfulfilled state and its beauty cannot shine through.

So much has been said and written about exercise and its benefits, but the most important thing is so often left out. Exercise must be done with joy to be effective! One of the most joyful ways to exercise is to dance. As women, we were made to dance and rejoice - this is what your body secretly wants to do. Listen to your body and release that inner dancer!

Belly dancing is an art that has been practiced and refined for a very long time in the Middle East. It is beautiful to watch and it will reshape your body, making you the woman you were designed to be. It is a joyful art form and most teachers of this ancient exercise insist that you smile when you are practicing and performing. I say this: it is difficult not to smile when you are expressing yourself through this wonderful art form.

Belly dancing brings you all the benefits of a standard exercise program: cardiovascular rejuvenation, muscle toning and development of the body core. But it does so in a way that develops your muscles is a feminine way, adding not manly bulk but womanly curves.

Belly dancing is also a wonderful low-impact regimen for all of your joints, especially your spine. It increases their flexibility and range of motion and it teaches each of them to move gracefully.

It also increases your confidence in a wonderful and thoroughly self-affirming way.

You need to get yourself some belly dancing videos so you can practice every day at home and you need to enroll in a local class.

Make your home dance sessions a special time of beauty. Do them when and where you will not be disturbed by phones or family. I light a scented candle before I begin because it helps to set this time apart for me. I blow it out and put it away when I am finished. Before you dance, you should shower, put on light perfume and jewelry and a beautiful belly dancing outfit. No sweats or shorts for this!

In some areas you will find many belly dance schools listed on the internet. If so, visit several and find one that has a joyful and accepting atmosphere. And it is important that they do recitals. If there are none nearby, consider doing a bit of travel. A 45-minute drive is not too much if that's what it takes to find this joyful experience.

While belly dancing is best, there are also many forms of folk dancing which you can do. Israeli, Greek, Irish and others are terrific choices because of their gracefulness and exuberance.

As for other exercises, I recommend walking outdoors, but only in beautiful places that make you feel beautiful. No city streets with exhaust fumes, no bleak industrial areas. Choose lovely parks, exhilarating beaches, fragrant forests and sunny meadows. Bathe yourself in the sounds of nature: enjoy the birds, the sound of the wing blowing through the trees – all the natural music that was put there for you. Now I'm not against taking a long a little manmade music now and then, but I believe it is best if you avoid anything that strikes you as harsh, angry or violent.

Other good places to walk are amusement parks, malls and zoos! A family outing (or an afternoon with friends) can double as exercise and everyone will be happy.

A really good walk should be about an hour, but even a short walk is very beneficial. Find hidden opportunities for walks. For example, how about, every now and then when you go shopping, park at the far end of the lot and enjoy the walk up to the store. If you dare, smile at people as you go.

4 About Your Skin

You are what you eat!

A few years ago, authorities were telling us that food had no effect on the health of the skin. What tragic results that had for some of us. The tide has now turned and now, more and more health care professionals are recognizing the connection.

If you are not happy about your skin, seek the help of a dermatologist, a dietician, and herbalist or one of the few biochemists who are in private practice. They can be very helpful, but they are only human and if you're not satisfied, I recommend you experiment on your own. Try varying your diet and see what effect it has on the skin. You can begin by eliminating certain foods or food groups and see what you learn.

When I was a teenager and in my twenties, I was plagued by acne. After trying numerous treatments, I learned through trial and error, that if I simply eliminated gluten, caffeine and dairy products, my skin would become not just smooth and healthy, but radiant.

<u>Baby your skin with natural salves you can make at home</u>

<u>{Tommi – talk about benezenite clay, honey, etc.}</u>

<u>Also mention that product you use</u>

5 The Importance of Posture: Take a Stand

Your body tells the word a story by its posture. When a person slumps over, their body conveys sadness, old age and discouragement. When they stand up straight, they tell a story of joy, energy, youth and success.

Try this experiment. Put yourself in a public place and observe people's posture. Notice how different they all are! Now focus for just a moment on someone whose posture is not so good. Imagine how they would look if they were standing tall.

Good posture makes you beautiful in more than one way. It helps you project the positive energy that is your birthright and it also makes you healthier … and we all know that a healthy body is a beautiful body. Without going into more detail than you need right now, good posture makes more room for the bodily organs to work properly. The heart, lungs and digestive system in particular benefit from standing up properly.

Some women go to modeling schools to learn proper posture and get excellent results. There is

also something very effective that you can do
yourself at home:

1. Imagine that your head is a helium-filled
   balloon and it is rising, trying to pull your
   body upward. Feel you back straighten up
   and your chest expand. You may well be
   standing an inch or two taller at this point,
   making you look leaner and more graceful.
2. Look at yourself in a full-length mirror. As
   always, first say "Hello beautiful lady!"
   Then take a close look at your shoulders.
   Are they even? For most of us the answer is
   "no." Do what you can to even them up.
   Looks a lot better, doesn't it?
3. Maintain this stance for a little longer each
   day. It won't take long to develop the
   muscles required to do it automatically.

Tip: If you carry a shoulder bag, don't always put it
on the same side of your body as that can foster
uneven muscle development. However, if one of
your shoulders droops, place the bag on that
shoulder more often than the other to strengthen it.

6 Nutrition – Eat Like You Mean It

There is so much information out there on healthy eating that I hate to add more but I will make a few general comments.

First, eat like you mean it! That is to say, you need to create or buy meals that are beautiful to you and that you will heartily enjoy eating. That will, of course, vary widely from one person to another.

General principles:

One, use lemon water and carbonated water as I suggested in Chapter 1. You will be glad you did!

Two, watch your sodium intake carefully. Excess sodium can cause a variety of health and beauty problems, not the least of which is high blood pressure. In addition to making a person more prone to stroke and heart disease and other serious conditions, high blood pressure can cause unnatural reddening of the face which is a sad detriment to beauty. Beyond this, some medicines that are used to treat high blood pressure can have side effects. That being said, do never self-adjust your blood pressure meds without consulting your doctor.

Some women choose to eliminate salt completely from their diets and this is something you might want to consider if you have ever had a blood pressure issue. You will find that citrus juices, vinegar and spices make delicious substitutes for salt, often bringing out a very different characters in familiar dishes. Salt-free cooking also brings out a subtle sweetness in many foods that once tasted is hard to resist.

There are some people who mistakenly believe that soy sauce is somehow healthier than table salt. This is absolutely not the case. There are also some who think that sea salt has less sodium and this too is false.

Three, limit your consumption of sugar. In most people, excess sugar causes the belly to swell which is detrimental to your beauty and your posture. You may be surprised how quickly "sugar belly" goes away when you cut down your consumption of sweets.

Never drink sugar! A can of soda pop contains far more sugar than you might imagine. Just compare the nutritional information with other sweet foods.

Four, for lovely feminine curves, eat plenty of vegetables. The phytoestrogens they contain help round the breasts and other key body areas.

Five, make variety a key part of your diet. It will keep you focused on the enjoyability of the food you eat rather than on the quantity. In particular, rotate through lots of different vegetables and spices to make sure you get the benefits of each.

Six, include the foods listed below as they are believed to prevent vascularization of unwanted growths:

- Oily cold-water fish such as sardines and salmon
- Bok choy (a delicious Chinese cabbage relative)
- Berries
- Artichoke hearts
- Cooked tomatoes

Seven, tame the appetite monster!

When you sit down to a meal, whether you prepared it or someone else did, your appetite is a snarling beast. "Eat hearty! Eat big!" it orders you.

Here's how to reduce that snarl to a purr. In the first few minutes of a meal (or just before the meal) eat three things: something warm, something cold and something sweet. The cold can be your carbonated water, the warm can be a clear soup (chicken soup and vegetable soup are great), and the sweet can be a handful of berries or some other fruit. You will find that your desire to "eat hearty and eat big" has greatly diminished. Hooray!

Whether you are at a table or at a buffet, fill your plate once and only once. Pile it as high as you like, but never, ever accept seconds. If you're at a buffet-style restaurant go to the serving area one time only.

Eight. If you've done all the things I've suggested to you above, go ahead and have some dessert. If you can, that it is! Chances are, you will not be in the mood for anything resembling desert. And if you are, you will probably not be in the mood to eat much of it.

7 Accentuate Your Beauty with Color

6 The meaning of GLOW

As women, we need to love our sisters and that is
why I wrote this book.

Youth is not based on how old a woman is; it's an
energy we radiate when we are healthy and fulfilled.
It's an energy which projects love and assurance to
those around us. To me, the source of that energy is
God as revealed in the ancient Holy Scriptures
which are today called the Bible.

Others may have different sources of inspiration:
nature, music, art, etc. In spite of these differences,
I believe we are all on the same spiritual path. If we
traverse that path in honesty and purity, rejecting all
that we find false and all things that are destructive
to ourselves or others, then I believe we will
eventually be drawn to Yeshua the Messiah, known
in English as Jesus the Christ.

Men are attracted by our beauty, but that's not why

we develop ourselves. We live to be fulfilled and if,
for you, fulfillment includes earthly love, then your
GLOW and your beauty will be a great asset in
achieving it.

Beauty is not just how we look, all though that is
without doubt a part of it. Beauty is also about
what's going on inside our minds and hearts. To
have a beautiful day, we must begin by taking care
of our bodies, but we must also attend to our
thoughts and feelings. Are you harboring anger
against someone who has wronged you? Give it up.
Forgive them although they may not deserve it. As
the popular song says, "The jury and the judge say
you've got a right to hold a grudge, but forgive
them." You will be the one who reaps the greatest
benefits.

Forgiveness is no easier to accomplish than any of
the other advice I give in this book, but if you work
on it, you will achieve it. If you ask God to help
you, He will make it much easier for you.

Get rid of any plans or fantasies you may have
about getting revenge of any kind. These thought
patterns are destructive to your beauty by robbing
you of inner peace. I'm certainly not saying you
should stay in abusive relationships or that you
should not avoid people you know want to do you
mental, physical or spiritual harm. Do what you
need to do to protect yourself, but keep your inner

soul from entanglement.

9 What Comes Next?

There's nothing more energizing than seeing your progress on paper or on your computer!

 It's best if you can start Day 1.

- Make a chart, wither on paper or electronically. Take your measurements and weigh yourself and enter the numbers on the chart.

- Update the chart each week.

When your friends start asking why you are looking so good, don't keep it a secret! Tell them about this little book and let them become your partners in beauty.

I'd love to hear about your progress!

Just send me an email at tommipabst@yahoo.com.

10

Additional Support for Your Weight Loss and Beauty Program

If you want to purchase any of the items I mention in this book, they will soon be available on our website!

If you would like to receive a detailed plan book covering exactly what to do each month, you will be able to find that on the website, too.

I offer in-depth GLOW counseling in several formats:

- On-line seminars using Skype or similar software.
- Group seminars at your U.S., European, Asian or Australian location.

These seminars are all about making the GLOW weight loss and beauty plan work for you! Please choose from the following topics:

- The GLOW weight loss plan
- The GLOW skin care plan

- The GLOW exercise plan
- The GLOW posture plan
- The GLOW fashion and color sense plan

I also offer private on-line help sessions and private consultation in your home.

Please call the GLOW hotline for pricing and scheduling information. 513-557-1938.

Remember – you can and will reach your goals!